Mom to Be: Quick Guide for Breastfeeding

LM Glenn

Published by LM Glenn, 2024.

While every precaution has been taken in the preparation of this book, the publisher assumes no responsibility for errors or omissions, or for damages resulting from the use of the information contained herein.

MOM TO BE: QUICK GUIDE FOR BREASTFEEDING

First edition. August 9, 2024.

Copyright © 2024 LM Glenn.

ISBN: 979-8227212207

Written by LM Glenn.

Section I: Introduction to Breastfeeding and Common Misconceptions

Introduction to Breastfeeding:

Breastfeeding is one of the most natural and beneficial practices a mother can offer her newborn. It provides essential nutrients, fosters a unique bond between mother and child, and offers numerous health benefits for both parties. The World Health Organization (WHO) and the American Academy of Pediatrics (AAP) recommend exclusive breastfeeding for the first six months of a baby's life, followed by continued breastfeeding along with the introduction of complementary foods for up to two years or beyond. These recommendations are rooted in extensive research showing that breastfeeding can significantly reduce the risk of infections, chronic conditions, and even certain types of cancer for both mother and child.

However, despite these well-documented benefits, many women struggle with breastfeeding. In some cases, these struggles are due to physical challenges or lack of support, but often, they stem from widespread misconceptions that can shape expectations and experiences. Misconceptions about breastfeeding can lead to unnecessary stress, feelings of failure, and in some cases, premature weaning. Understanding and addressing these misconceptions is crucial for empowering mothers to make informed decisions about feeding their babies and to seek the support they need to succeed.

Common Misconceptions Overview:

Misconceptions about breastfeeding are pervasive and can vary widely depending on cultural, societal, and even familial influences. Some myths may be based on outdated information, while others are simply misunderstandings that have been perpetuated over time. These misconceptions can have a profound impact on a mother's breastfeeding journey, influencing her confidence, comfort, and ultimately, her decision to continue or stop breastfeeding.

In this book, we will explore some of the most common misconceptions surrounding breastfeeding, examining the truth behind these myths and their potential impact on mothers and babies. By dispelling these misconceptions, we aim to provide a clearer understanding of breastfeeding, highlighting the importance of accurate information and supportive environments for all mothers.

Misconception 1 – Breastfeeding is Easy and Natural for Everyone

The Myth:

One of the most common misconceptions is the belief that breastfeeding is a natural process that should come easily to all mothers and babies. Many assume that because breastfeeding is a biological function, it will naturally occur without any challenges. This belief is often reinforced by media portrayals of serene mothers effortlessly nursing their babies, creating an unrealistic expectation for many women.

The Reality:

While breastfeeding is a natural process, it is not always easy. In fact, many new mothers encounter various challenges that can make breastfeeding difficult. Common issues include difficulties with latching, low milk supply, nipple pain, and engorgement. For some mothers, these challenges can be overwhelming, especially if they are not prepared for the possibility that breastfeeding may not go as smoothly as they hoped.

The reality is that breastfeeding is a skill that both mother and baby need to learn together. It often takes time, patience, and practice to get it right. For some, it may take days or even weeks before breastfeeding becomes comfortable and routine. This is why support from lactation consultants, healthcare providers, and breastfeeding support groups is so crucial. These resources can provide guidance, tips, and reassurance that the challenges faced are normal and can be overcome with the right support.

Impact on Mothers:

The misconception that breastfeeding should be easy can have a significant emotional impact on mothers. When faced with challenges, many women may feel like they are failing or that something is wrong with them. This can lead to feelings of inadequacy, frustration, and even postpartum depression. Some mothers may be tempted to give up breastfeeding altogether, believing that they are not capable of doing it "right."

It is essential to normalize the idea that breastfeeding can be challenging, and that seeking help is not only okay but encouraged. By dispelling the myth that breastfeeding is always easy, we can help mothers feel more prepared and supported, reducing the pressure they may feel to be perfect from the start.

Misconception 2 – Formula is Just as Good as Breast Milk

The Myth:

Another prevalent misconception is the belief that formula is an equivalent or even superior substitute for breast milk. This myth is often fueled by aggressive marketing from formula companies, coupled with the idea that modern science can create products that mimic the nutritional profile of breast milk. Some parents may also believe that formula feeding is more convenient, consistent, or reliable than breastfeeding.

The Reality:

While infant formula is a safe and viable alternative for babies who cannot be breastfed, it is not equivalent to breast milk. Breast milk is a living fluid, rich in antibodies, enzymes, hormones, and growth factors that cannot be replicated in formula. It is uniquely tailored to meet the changing nutritional needs of the baby, providing not only optimal nutrition but also protection against infections, allergies, and chronic conditions like obesity and diabetes.

Breastfeeding also offers significant benefits for mothers, including a reduced risk of certain cancers, cardiovascular disease, and postpartum depression. The act of breastfeeding promotes bonding between mother and baby, releasing hormones like oxytocin that foster a sense of connection and well-being.

It's important to acknowledge that formula feeding can be necessary and beneficial in certain situations, such as when a mother is unable to produce enough milk or when breastfeeding is contraindicated due to health reasons. However, the decision to use formula should be informed by a clear understanding of the differences between formula and breast milk, rather than misconceptions about their equivalence.

Impact on Feeding Choices:

The misconception that formula is just as good as breast milk can lead some mothers to choose formula feeding without fully understanding the unique benefits of breastfeeding. This decision may be made out of convenience or a belief that formula will provide the same nutritional and health benefits as breast milk. While formula can be a lifesaver in certain situations, it's important for mothers to have access to accurate information so they can make informed choices that best suit their needs and those of their babies.

Healthcare providers play a crucial role in educating parents about the benefits of breastfeeding and offering support to those who wish to breastfeed. By addressing this misconception, we can help ensure that mothers who want to breastfeed feel confident and supported in their decision, while also respecting the choices of those who opt for formula.

Misconception 3 – You Must Stop Breastfeeding When Returning to Work

The Myth:

A common misconception among working mothers is the belief that they must stop breastfeeding when they return to work. This myth is often rooted in concerns about the logistics of pumping, storing milk, and maintaining a breastfeeding schedule while balancing the demands of a job. Some women may also fear that their workplace will not be supportive of their breastfeeding needs.

The Reality:

The reality is that many working mothers successfully continue breastfeeding after returning to work, thanks to strategies like pumping and storing breast milk. With proper planning and support, it is entirely possible to maintain a breastfeeding relationship while working outside the home.

Legal protections, such as the Affordable Care Act in the United States, require employers to provide reasonable break times and a private, non-bathroom space for breastfeeding mothers to pump. These provisions make it easier for mothers to continue breastfeeding, even in demanding work environments.

Many workplaces are increasingly recognizing the importance of supporting breastfeeding mothers, offering lactation rooms, flexible schedules, and resources to help ease the transition back to work. It's important for mothers to communicate their needs with their employers and to seek out workplace support, whether through human resources, employee assistance programs, or peer networks.

Impact on Working Mothers:

The misconception that breastfeeding and working are incompatible can cause significant stress and anxiety for new mothers. Some may feel pressured to wean their babies before they are ready or to switch to formula feeding, even if they would prefer to continue breastfeeding. This can lead to feelings of guilt, disappointment, and loss.

By dispelling this myth, we can empower working mothers to explore all their options and find solutions that work for their unique situations. Whether it's arranging for on-site childcare, coordinating pumping schedules, or negotiating flexible work arrangements, there are many ways to continue breastfeeding while pursuing a fulfilling career.

Misconception 4 – Breastfeeding is Painful and Causes Sagging Breasts

The Myth:

One of the more pervasive and fear-inducing misconceptions is the belief that breastfeeding is inherently painful and will lead to long-term physical changes, such as sagging breasts. This myth can deter some women from even attempting to breastfeed, out of fear that it will cause them discomfort or alter their bodies in undesirable ways.

The Reality:

While it is true that some discomfort can occur during the early stages of breastfeeding, persistent pain is not normal and should be addressed. Common causes of pain include improper latch, tongue-tie in the baby, or nipple trauma. These issues can often be resolved with the help of a lactation consultant or healthcare provider, allowing mothers to breastfeed comfortably.

As for the fear of sagging breasts, research has shown that breastfeeding is not the primary cause. Factors such as genetics, age, weight changes, and the number of pregnancies a woman has had play a much larger role in the natural changes that occur to the breasts over time. In fact, the changes that happen during pregnancy, when the breasts increase in size and prepare for lactation, are more likely to contribute to sagging than breastfeeding itself.

Impact on Breastfeeding Duration:

The fear of pain and body changes can lead some women to avoid breastfeeding altogether or to wean earlier than they might have otherwise. This misconception can deprive both mother and baby of the benefits of breastfeeding and contribute to negative feelings about the postpartum body.

It is important to provide accurate information and reassurance to expectant and new mothers. Breastfeeding should not be painful, and any discomfort can often be alleviated with the right support. Additionally, normalizing the natural **changes that** occur in a woman's body after pregnancy and breastfeeding can help reduce the stigma and fear associated with these changes.

Conclusion and Encouragement for Informed Breastfeeding Choices

We have explored some of the most common misconceptions surrounding breastfeeding, including the belief that breastfeeding is easy for everyone, that formula is equivalent to breast milk, that breastfeeding must stop when returning to work, and that breastfeeding is painful and causes sagging breasts. Each of these myths has the potential to impact a mother's breastfeeding journey, influencing her decisions, her confidence, and her overall experience.

Encouragement for Support and Education:

It is vital for mothers to have access to accurate information and support throughout their breastfeeding journey. Healthcare providers, lactation consultants, and breastfeeding support groups play a crucial role in educating mothers and helping them navigate any challenges they may face. By dispelling these misconceptions, we can create a more supportive environment for breastfeeding, where mothers feel empowered to make the best choices for themselves and their babies.

Final Thoughts:

Breastfeeding is a deeply personal and unique experience for each mother and baby. What works for one family may not work for another, and that's okay. The most important thing is that mothers feel informed, supported, and confident in their feeding choices, whether they choose to breastfeed, use formula, or a combination of both. By addressing and correcting common misconceptions, we can help ensure that every mother has the knowledge and resources she needs to make the best decision for her family.

Section II: Guide to Breastfeeding

Breastfeeding is a natural and beneficial way to nourish your baby, but it can also come with its own set of challenges and questions. This guide is designed to help new moms who choose to breastfeed by providing essential information, tips, and encouragement.

I. Benefits of Breastfeeding

- **For Baby:**
    - Provides ideal nutrition, perfectly balanced for a baby's needs.
    - Boosts the immune system and helps protect against infections.
    - Reduces the risk of sudden infant death syndrome (SIDS).
    - Promotes healthy weight and reduces the risk of childhood obesity.
    - Encourages proper jaw and teeth development.
- **For Mom:**
    - Helps the uterus contract, reducing postpartum bleeding.
    - Burns extra calories, aiding in postpartum weight loss.
    - Lowers the risk of breast and ovarian cancers.
    - Strengthens the bond between mother and baby.
    - Saves money and time compared to formula feeding.

II. Preparing for Breastfeeding

- **Education:**
    - Take a breastfeeding class before delivery to learn about techniques and what to expect.

- Read books and reputable online resources to familiarize yourself with breastfeeding basics.
- **Gathering Supplies:**
  - Nursing bras and pads for comfort and leakage management.
  - A good breast pump if you plan to express milk.
  - Breastfeeding pillows to help position your baby comfortably.
  - Storage bags for expressed milk if you plan to pump.
- **Setting Up a Nursing Space:**
  - Choose a quiet, comfortable spot with supportive seating.
  - Keep essentials like water, snacks, burp cloths, and entertainment (books, TV remote) within reach.

III. The First Few Days

- **Initiating Breastfeeding:**
  - Begin breastfeeding within the first hour after birth if possible. This helps establish milk supply and promotes bonding.
  - Skin-to-skin contact is important to stimulate your baby's natural feeding instincts.
- **Colostrum:**
  - Your first milk is colostrum, a thick, yellowish substance rich in nutrients and antibodies.
  - It's normal to produce only a small amount; this is all your baby needs in the first few days.
- **Frequency of Feeding:**
  - Newborns typically feed 8-12 times in 24 hours.
  - Follow your baby's hunger cues (rooting, sucking motions) rather than a strict schedule.

- **Latching On:**
  - Ensure your baby's mouth covers both the nipple and part of the areola.
  - A good latch is key to preventing pain and ensuring efficient milk transfer.
  - If you experience discomfort, gently break the latch by inserting a clean finger into the corner of your baby's mouth and try again.

IV. Establishing Milk Supply

- **Frequent Nursing:**
  - Breastfeed often to stimulate milk production, as milk supply works on a supply-and-demand basis.
- **Hydration and Nutrition:**
  - Drink plenty of water and eat a balanced diet to support your milk supply.
  - Include foods rich in vitamins, minerals, and healthy fats.
- **Pumping:**
  - Pumping can help maintain or increase milk supply, especially if you are separated from your baby.
  - Pump after feeding if you need to increase supply or if your baby isn't nursing effectively.
- **Rest and Self-Care:**
  - Rest as much as possible to help your body recover and produce milk.
  - Accept help with household tasks and focus on bonding with your baby.

V. Overcoming Common Challenges

- **Sore Nipples:**
    - Ensure a proper latch to minimize nipple pain.
    - Apply lanolin cream or breast milk to soothe sore nipples.
    - Air-dry nipples after feeding and wear loose-fitting clothing.
- **Engorgement:**
    - Feed frequently or express milk to relieve engorgement.
    - Apply warm compresses before feeding and cold compresses after to reduce swelling.
- **Blocked Ducts and Mastitis:**
    - Massage the breast gently toward the nipple while feeding.
    - Continue breastfeeding even if you have mastitis but consult a doctor if you have symptoms like fever and chills.
- **Low Milk Supply:**
    - Nurse or pump more frequently to stimulate production.
    - Consider lactation aids like fenugreek or consult a lactation specialist.
- **Inverted or Flat Nipples:**
    - Use a nipple shield or try techniques like the Hoffman exercise to help your baby latch.

VI. Breastfeeding in Different Situations

- **Breastfeeding in Public:**
    - Practice at home to gain confidence and use a nursing cover if you prefer privacy.
    - Know your rights regarding breastfeeding in public.

- **Returning to Work:**
  - ○ Discuss your pumping needs with your employer and establish a routine for pumping at work.
  - ○ Build a milk stash by pumping after morning feedings a few weeks before returning to work.
- **Breastfeeding Twins or Multiples:**
  - ○ Tandem feeding (nursing two babies at once) can save time.
  - ○ Consider using a breastfeeding pillow designed for twins.
- **Breastfeeding with a Health Condition:**
  - ○ Many health conditions are compatible with breastfeeding but consult your doctor.
  - ○ Some medications are safe during breastfeeding; always check with a healthcare provider.

VII. Weaning and Transitioning

- **When to Wean:**
  - ○ Weaning can be gradual and should be based on you and your baby's needs.
  - ○ Some mothers wean at 6 months, while others continue breastfeeding into toddlerhood.
- **How to Wean:**
  - ○ Drop one feeding at a time, starting with the least preferred.
  - ○ Replace breastfeeding with other comforts like cuddling or reading.
- **Emotional Aspects:**
  - ○ Weaning can be an emotional process; it's normal to feel a mix of sadness and relief.
  - ○ Focus on the new ways you can bond with your child.

VIII. Support and Resources

- **Lactation Consultants:**
    - Seek help from a lactation consultant if you encounter difficulties or need personalized advice.
- **Breastfeeding Support Groups:**
    - Joining a local or online breastfeeding group can provide encouragement and a sense of community.
- **Helplines and Websites:**
    - Utilize resources like the La Leche League or local breastfeeding hotlines for immediate support.

IX. Frequently Asked Questions

- **Is my baby getting enough milk?**
    - Look for signs like steady weight gain, contentment after feeding, and regular wet and dirty diapers.
- **How long should each feeding last?**
    - Newborns may nurse for 20-45 minutes. As they grow, feedings may become shorter.
- **Can I breastfeed if I'm sick?**
    - In most cases, breastfeeding is safe and beneficial even when you're ill. Your antibodies can help protect your baby.

X. Final Thoughts and Encouragement

- **Patience and Persistence:**
    - Breastfeeding can take time to master, so be patient with yourself and your baby.

- **Celebrate Small Wins:**
    - ○ Every day you breastfeed is a success. Take pride in providing your baby with the best start in life.
- **Trust Your Instincts:**
    - ○ You know your baby better than anyone else. Trust your instincts and do what feels right for both of you.

Breastfeeding is a unique and personal journey. Remember, it's okay to seek help, and it's okay to make decisions that work best for you and your family. You're doing a wonderful job, and every drop of breast milk you provide is a gift to your baby.

Section III: Nutritional Benefits to Breastfeeding

Introduction

Breastfeeding has been a fundamental practice since the dawn of humanity, playing a crucial role in the survival and development of infants. It is not only a natural way to nourish newborns but also a deeply embedded cultural practice that has been valued across civilizations for millennia. Today, the significance of breastfeeding is underscored by extensive scientific research, which highlights its myriad health benefits. In an era where alternatives such as formula feeding are readily available, it is essential to understand the unique advantages that breastfeeding offers. These benefits extend beyond basic nutrition, influencing both the immediate and long-term health of the child, the well-being of the mother, and even the economic and public health landscape. This essay will explore the comprehensive health benefits of breastfeeding, demonstrating why it remains the gold standard for infant nutrition and maternal health.

Nutritional Benefits for Infants

One of the most significant advantages of breastfeeding is the unparalleled nutritional value of breast milk. Breast milk is a complex and dynamic fluid, uniquely tailored to meet the nutritional needs of the infant. Unlike formula, which is a static product, breast milk changes in composition over time, adapting to the growing and changing needs of the baby. During the first few days postpartum, the mother produces colostrum, a thick, yellowish fluid that is rich in antibodies and low in fat, providing essential nutrients and immune protection to the newborn. As the infant grows, the composition of breast milk shifts to meet their nutritional needs, offering the perfect balance of fats, proteins, and carbohydrates.

Breast milk is also more easily digested by infants compared to formula. This ease of digestion is crucial for a newborn's developing digestive system, which is not yet fully matured. The natural enzymes present in breast milk, such as lipase, help to break down fats, making it easier for the infant to absorb essential nutrients. Additionally, breast milk contains oligosaccharides, a type of carbohydrate that promotes the growth of healthy gut bacteria, further supporting the infant's digestive health.

Immune System Support for Infants

Beyond its nutritional value, breast milk plays a vital role in bolstering the infant's immune system. It contains a variety of immune-boosting components, including antibodies, white blood cells, and lactoferrin, all of which help protect the infant from infections and diseases. The presence of immunoglobulin A (IgA) in breast milk is particularly important, as it coats the lining of the infant's intestines, preventing harmful pathogens from entering the bloodstream.

Breastfed infants are less likely to suffer from common childhood illnesses, such as respiratory infections, ear infections, and gastrointestinal disturbances. The protective effects of breastfeeding are so significant that they extend well beyond the breastfeeding period, offering long-term immunity benefits. Studies have shown that breastfed children have lower rates of chronic conditions, such as asthma, allergies, and autoimmune diseases, compared to their formula-fed counterparts.

Cognitive and Developmental Advantages

Breastfeeding has also been linked to enhanced cognitive development in children. The essential fatty acids found in breast milk, particularly docosahexaenoic acid (DHA) and arachidonic acid (ARA), are critical for brain development. These nutrients are abundant in breast milk but are often lacking in formula, even though some formulas are fortified with DHA and ARA, they do not replicate the natural balance found in breast milk.

Research indicates that children who are breastfed tend to score higher on IQ tests and perform better academically than those who are formula-fed. These cognitive benefits are believed to be due to the combination of essential nutrients and the close physical and emotional contact that breastfeeding provides. The act of breastfeeding also promotes the development of social and emotional skills, as the infant learns to interact and bond with the mother during feeding.

Health Benefits for Mothers

Breastfeeding is not only beneficial for infants but also offers significant health advantages for mothers. One of the immediate benefits is the role breastfeeding plays in postpartum recovery. The hormone oxytocin, released during breastfeeding, helps the uterus contract and return to its pre-pregnancy size more quickly, reducing the risk of postpartum hemorrhage. Additionally, breastfeeding can delay the return of menstruation, acting as a natural form of birth control during the first six months postpartum, provided that breastfeeding is exclusive and the mother has not yet resumed her menstrual cycle.

In the long term, breastfeeding has been associated with a reduced risk of developing breast and ovarian cancers. The hormonal changes induced by breastfeeding are thought to lower estrogen levels, thereby reducing the risk of hormone-related cancers. Moreover, breastfeeding has been linked to a lower risk of osteoporosis and cardiovascular diseases later in life. These protective effects increase with the duration of breastfeeding, making it a vital practice for long-term maternal health.

Conclusion

In conclusion, breastfeeding is a practice with profound health benefits for both infants and mothers. From providing optimal nutrition and immune protection to promoting cognitive development and reducing the risk of chronic diseases, the advantages of breastfeeding are far-reaching. Additionally, breastfeeding contributes to the emotional well-being of both mother and child, fostering a strong bond that enhances mental health. The societal and economic benefits further underscore the importance of supporting and promoting breastfeeding as a public health priority. Given the extensive evidence supporting the health benefits of breastfeeding, it is essential to educate parents and provide the necessary support to ensure that breastfeeding is accessible and feasible for all families.

Section IV: Role of Healthcare Provider

Breastfeeding is a critical public health issue, offering extensive benefits for both infants and mothers. These benefits are well-documented and include nutritional superiority, enhanced immunity, and emotional bonding. Despite this, global breastfeeding rates remain below optimal levels, with many mothers encountering significant barriers to breastfeeding successfully. Healthcare providers and policies play an instrumental role in either facilitating or hindering breastfeeding practices. The involvement of healthcare providers—ranging from obstetricians and midwives to pediatricians and lactation consultants—is crucial in educating, supporting, and encouraging mothers to initiate and continue breastfeeding. At the same time, supportive policies, both at the institutional and governmental levels, are essential to create an environment where breastfeeding is normalized and supported. This essay will delve into the pivotal role of healthcare providers in promoting breastfeeding and examine the impact of policies that support this practice, highlighting their significance in improving public health outcomes.

The Importance of Breastfeeding

Breastfeeding is widely recognized as the best source of nutrition for infants, offering a perfect balance of nutrients that are easily digestible and perfectly suited to the needs of a growing baby. Breast milk provides the necessary antibodies to protect infants from a variety of infections, reducing the incidence of respiratory illnesses, ear infections, and gastrointestinal problems. Moreover, breastfeeding has been associated with long-term benefits, including reduced risks of chronic conditions such as obesity, type 2 diabetes, and certain types of cancer. For mothers, breastfeeding helps in postpartum recovery, reduces the risk of breast and ovarian cancers, and promotes emotional bonding with the infant.

The economic benefits of breastfeeding are also significant, reducing healthcare costs by lowering the rates of infant illness and hospitalization and decreasing the need for expensive formula. These factors underline the importance of breastfeeding as a public health priority and the need for strong support systems to encourage and sustain breastfeeding practices.

Role of Healthcare Providers

Healthcare providers are at the forefront of breastfeeding promotion, acting as trusted sources of information and support for new mothers. Their role begins during pregnancy, where they can educate expectant mothers about the benefits of breastfeeding and prepare them for the challenges they may face. Midwives and obstetricians are often the first to introduce the concept of breastfeeding and can offer valuable guidance on its importance.

Once the baby is born, healthcare providers play a crucial role in initiating breastfeeding. Early initiation, ideally within the first hour after birth, is strongly associated with longer breastfeeding duration and greater breastfeeding success. In hospital settings, lactation consultants and nurses provide hands-on support to ensure that mothers are comfortable and confident in breastfeeding their newborns. This support is vital, especially in the early days when mothers may encounter difficulties such as latching problems or concerns about milk supply.

Continued support from healthcare providers after the mother and baby leave the hospital is equally important. Pediatricians, family doctors, and community health nurses can monitor the baby's growth, address any breastfeeding concerns, and encourage mothers to continue breastfeeding for as long as possible. The role of healthcare providers in this ongoing support cannot be overstated, as they are often the first point of contact when mothers encounter challenges that may lead to early cessation of breastfeeding.

Challenges Faced by Healthcare Providers

Despite their critical role, healthcare providers often face significant challenges in promoting breastfeeding. One major barrier is the lack of adequate training and education on breastfeeding practices. Many healthcare professionals receive limited instruction on breastfeeding during their formal education, which can leave them ill-equipped to address the complexities of breastfeeding management.

Time constraints and heavy workloads also pose challenges. In busy hospital environments, healthcare providers may not have the time to offer the necessary support and encouragement to breastfeeding mothers. This is particularly problematic in settings where staff shortages are common, and the demand for care is high.

Cultural and social barriers can further complicate the promotion of breastfeeding. In some communities, there may be stigma or misinformation surrounding breastfeeding, making it difficult for healthcare providers to advocate for it effectively. Additionally, conflicting information from various sources, including the internet and social networks, can undermine the advice given by healthcare professionals, leading to confusion and doubt among new mothers.

Policies Promoting Breastfeeding

Effective policies are essential to support healthcare providers in promoting breastfeeding and to create an environment where breastfeeding is encouraged and supported at all levels of society. National and international guidelines, such as those from the World Health Organization (WHO) and UNICEF, provide a framework for breastfeeding promotion. These guidelines advocate for practices such as the early initiation of breastfeeding, exclusive breastfeeding for the first six months, and continued breastfeeding along with appropriate complementary foods up to two years of age or beyond.

Legislation plays a critical role in supporting breastfeeding, particularly in terms of maternity leave policies and workplace accommodations. Laws that provide for paid maternity leave allow mothers the time they need to establish and maintain breastfeeding without the pressure of returning to work too soon. Workplace accommodations, such as providing time and space for breastfeeding or pumping, are also crucial in enabling mothers to continue breastfeeding after they return to work.

Public health campaigns and initiatives, such as the Baby-Friendly Hospital Initiative (BFHI), have been instrumental in promoting breastfeeding. The BFHI, launched by WHO and UNICEF, encourages hospitals to create environments that support breastfeeding, including the provision of rooming-in and breastfeeding support. The impact of such initiatives can be seen in the increased breastfeeding rates in hospitals that have implemented the BFHI.

Non-governmental organizations (NGOs) and advocacy groups also play a vital role in promoting breastfeeding through public education campaigns, lobbying for supportive legislation, and providing resources and support for breastfeeding mothers. These organizations often work in tandem with healthcare providers and policymakers to create a comprehensive support system for breastfeeding.

Case Studies and Success Stories

To understand the impact of healthcare providers and policies on breastfeeding promotion, it is useful to examine case studies and success stories from around the world. The Baby-Friendly Hospital Initiative, for example, has been highly successful in increasing breastfeeding rates in hospitals that have adopted its practices. Studies have shown that mothers who give birth in Baby-Friendly hospitals are more likely to initiate breastfeeding and continue breastfeeding exclusively for the recommended six months.

Countries with strong breastfeeding support systems, such as Norway and Sweden, have some of the highest breastfeeding rates in the world. These countries have implemented comprehensive maternity leave policies, extensive breastfeeding education for healthcare providers, and widespread public health campaigns that normalize and encourage breastfeeding. The success of these countries highlights the importance of a multifaceted approach that includes healthcare provider involvement, supportive policies, and public education.

Recommendations for Improvement

Despite the progress made in promoting breastfeeding, there is still much work to be done. One of the most important areas for improvement is the enhancement of training and resources for healthcare providers. Healthcare professionals need more comprehensive education on breastfeeding management, including how to address common challenges and provide effective support to mothers.

Strengthening policy enforcement is also crucial. While many countries have laws supporting breastfeeding, these laws are not always adequately enforced. For example, while maternity leave policies exist in many places, they are often not long enough, or employers may not fully comply with workplace accommodation requirements. Ensuring that these policies are enforced and creating new policies where gaps exist can significantly improve breastfeeding rates.

Community involvement and peer support groups are also essential in promoting breastfeeding. Mothers who have access to support from other breastfeeding mothers are more likely to continue breastfeeding. Encouraging the formation of peer support groups and integrating them into the healthcare system can provide mothers with the encouragement and assistance they need.

Finally, addressing disparities in breastfeeding support is critical. In many cases, marginalized communities have lower breastfeeding rates due to a lack of access to healthcare services, cultural barriers, or economic challenges. Targeted interventions that address these disparities are needed to ensure that all mothers have the opportunity to breastfeed.

Conclusion

In conclusion, the promotion of breastfeeding is a complex but vital public health issue that requires the involvement of both healthcare providers and supportive policies. Healthcare providers play a key role in educating and supporting mothers, from the prenatal period through the early years of a child's life. However, their efforts must be backed by strong policies that provide the necessary time, space, and support for breastfeeding. Through continued education, enforcement of supportive policies, and targeted interventions, we can improve breastfeeding rates and, in turn, enhance the health and well-being of mothers and children worldwide. The role of healthcare providers and policies is indispensable in this effort, making it essential for all stakeholders to work together to promote and support breastfeeding.

Section V: Societal and Economic Implications of Breastfeeding

Breastfeeding has far-reaching societal and economic implications that extend beyond the immediate health benefits for mothers and infants. These implications influence public health, economic stability, social norms, and even environmental sustainability. Understanding these broader impacts is crucial for policymakers, healthcare providers, and society as a whole.

1. Public Health Benefits

Breastfeeding contributes significantly to the overall health of populations. By providing optimal nutrition and immune protection, breastfeeding reduces the incidence of infectious diseases, such as diarrhea and pneumonia, which are major causes of infant mortality in many parts of the world. The reduction in illness among breastfed children decreases the burden on healthcare systems, leading to fewer hospital visits, lower healthcare costs, and less strain on medical resources.

Long-term, breastfeeding is associated with a lower risk of chronic diseases such as obesity, diabetes, and cardiovascular conditions. This not only enhances individual health outcomes but also contributes to a healthier population, reducing the prevalence of these costly diseases and the need for long-term medical care.

2. Economic Savings

Breastfeeding offers substantial economic savings at both the individual and societal levels. For families, breastfeeding eliminates the need to purchase formula, which can be a significant expense, especially for families in low-income settings. In contrast, breast milk is a natural, cost-effective source of nutrition that is readily available and requires no preparation or special equipment.

At the societal level, the economic benefits of breastfeeding are seen in reduced healthcare costs. As breastfeeding lowers the incidence of common childhood illnesses, it results in fewer doctor visits, hospitalizations, and prescriptions, all of which contribute to lowering healthcare expenditures. Studies have estimated that if breastfeeding rates were increased to recommended levels, millions of dollars could be saved annually in healthcare costs.

Additionally, breastfeeding supports maternal health, leading to fewer health complications for mothers, which in turn reduces the need for medical interventions and associated costs. This economic impact extends to the workplace, where healthier mothers and children result in lower absenteeism and increased productivity.

3. Social Norms and Gender Equality

Breastfeeding is deeply intertwined with social norms and gender roles. In societies where breastfeeding is widely practiced and supported, it is often seen as a natural and expected part of motherhood. However, in cultures where formula feeding has become normalized or where breastfeeding in public is stigmatized, mothers may face significant social pressure and barriers to breastfeeding.

Promoting breastfeeding can contribute to advancing gender equality by emphasizing the value of maternal roles and providing women with the support they need to breastfeed. Policies that support breastfeeding, such as paid maternity leave and workplace accommodations, help to alleviate the pressure on women to choose between breastfeeding and their careers. By creating an environment where breastfeeding is both supported and normalized, societies can foster greater gender equality and empower women to make the best choices for themselves and their families.

4. Environmental Impact

Breastfeeding has positive environmental implications as well. Breast milk is a renewable, sustainable resource that requires no packaging, transportation, or waste disposal, unlike formula, which has a significant environmental footprint. The production and distribution of formula involve the use of energy, water, and raw materials, as well as the generation of waste from packaging and expired products.

By reducing the demand for formula, breastfeeding contributes to lower greenhouse gas emissions and less waste, making it an environmentally friendly option. Promoting breastfeeding as part of a broader strategy for environmental sustainability can help reduce the ecological impact of infant feeding practices.

5. Long-Term Societal Benefits

The long-term societal benefits of breastfeeding are also significant. Children who are breastfed tend to have better cognitive outcomes, leading to improved educational performance and higher productivity in adulthood. This has implications for the future workforce and the overall economic growth of a society.

Furthermore, the practice of breastfeeding strengthens the bond between mother and child, contributing to the emotional and psychological well-being of both. This, in turn, can lead to stronger family units and more stable communities, which are the foundation of a healthy society.

Conclusion

In summary, breastfeeding has profound societal and economic implications that extend beyond the immediate health benefits for mothers and infants. It contributes to public health, generates economic savings, supports gender equality, reduces environmental impact, and fosters long-term societal well-being. Recognizing these broader implications is essential for promoting breastfeeding as a public health priority and for developing policies that support and normalize breastfeeding across all sectors of society.

Section VI: Challenges and Barriers to Breastfeeding

Breastfeeding is widely recognized as the best source of nutrition for infants, offering a myriad of benefits for both the child and the mother. It provides essential nutrients, strengthens the immune system, and fosters bonding between mother and child. Despite these advantages, many mothers face significant challenges and barriers that can impede their ability to breastfeed successfully. These challenges can be categorized into physical, psychological, socio-economic, and environmental factors, all of which contribute to the complex landscape of breastfeeding.

1. Physical Challenges

One of the primary barriers to breastfeeding is the range of physical challenges that mothers may encounter. These include:

a. Lactation Problems: Many new mothers experience difficulties with lactation, such as low milk supply, overproduction of milk, or blocked milk ducts. These issues can lead to frustration and discomfort, making breastfeeding a stressful experience.

b. Nipple Pain and Damage: Nipple pain, often caused by improper latching, cracked nipples, or infections like mastitis, is a common issue that can deter mothers from continuing to breastfeed. This pain can be severe and lead to early weaning if not properly managed.

c. Medical Conditions: Certain medical conditions, such as hormonal imbalances, breast surgery, or chronic illnesses, can interfere with a mother's ability to produce enough milk or breastfeed comfortably.

2. Psychological and Emotional Barriers

The psychological and emotional well-being of the mother plays a crucial role in the success of breastfeeding. Some of the key barriers in this area include:

a. Postpartum Depression: Mothers experiencing postpartum depression may find it difficult to engage in breastfeeding due to feelings of sadness, anxiety, and a lack of motivation. This mental health condition can severely impact a mother's ability to bond with her child and maintain a breastfeeding routine.

b. Stress and Anxiety: The demands of caring for a newborn, coupled with societal pressures to breastfeed, can create immense stress and anxiety. This emotional burden can affect milk production and make breastfeeding a challenging task for many mothers.

c. Body Image Issues: Some women struggle with body image issues related to breastfeeding, such as concerns about sagging breasts or changes in appearance. These concerns can lead to reluctance to breastfeed or early cessation.

3. Socio-Economic Barriers

Socio-economic factors significantly influence a mother's ability to breastfeed. These barriers are often systemic and can be difficult to overcome without proper support and resources:

a. Lack of Paid Maternity Leave: In many countries, the absence of paid maternity leave forces mothers to return to work shortly after childbirth. This early return can make it challenging to establish a breastfeeding routine, leading to reliance on formula feeding.

b. Inadequate Workplace Support: Even when mothers are able to return to work, many face workplaces that are not breastfeeding-friendly. Lack of private spaces for pumping, inflexible work schedules, and unsupportive employers can all hinder a mother's ability to continue breastfeeding.

c. Economic Constraints: Low-income mothers may face additional challenges, such as limited access to breastfeeding education and support services. The cost of breastfeeding supplies, such as breast pumps and nursing bras, can also be a financial burden for some families.

4. Environmental and Societal Barriers

The environment and societal attitudes towards breastfeeding play a significant role in shaping a mother's breastfeeding experience. Key barriers in this area include:

a. Social Stigma and Public Perception: Despite growing awareness of the benefits of breastfeeding, societal stigma and negative public perception still persist. Many mothers feel uncomfortable breastfeeding in public due to fear of judgment or harassment, which can lead to reduced breastfeeding frequency and early weaning.

b. Cultural Norms and Beliefs: In some cultures, breastfeeding may not be the norm, or there may be misconceptions about breastfeeding practices. Cultural beliefs about the role of women, body image, and infant feeding can all influence a mother's decision to breastfeed.

c. Lack of Education and Support: A lack of education and support from healthcare providers, family members, and the community can be a significant barrier to breastfeeding. Mothers may not receive adequate information about the benefits of breastfeeding, how to overcome challenges, or where to seek help if needed.

5. Healthcare System Barriers

The healthcare system itself can also pose challenges to breastfeeding:

a. Inconsistent Medical Advice: Mothers may receive conflicting advice from different healthcare providers regarding breastfeeding, leading to confusion and frustration. Consistent and evidence-based guidance is essential for successful breastfeeding.

b. Limited Access to Lactation Consultants: Lactation consultants play a vital role in supporting breastfeeding mothers. However, access to these professionals is often limited, especially in rural or underserved areas, leaving mothers without the necessary support to overcome breastfeeding challenges.

c. Hospital Practices: Certain hospital practices, such as routine separation of mother and baby after birth or the promotion of formula feeding, can interfere with early breastfeeding initiation and success.

Conclusion

Breastfeeding, while natural, is not always easy. The challenges and barriers faced by mothers are diverse and multifaceted, encompassing physical, psychological, socio-economic, environmental, and systemic factors. Addressing these barriers requires a comprehensive approach that includes education, support, and policy changes. By providing mothers with the resources and support they need, society can help ensure that more mothers are able to successfully breastfeed, benefiting both their health and the health of their children.

Section VII: Global Perspectives on Breastfeeding

Breastfeeding is a universal practice, but how it is perceived and supported varies significantly across different cultures and countries. The cultural, social, and policy environments of a nation profoundly influence the breastfeeding practices of its mothers. While some countries actively promote and support breastfeeding through comprehensive public health policies and societal norms, others may struggle with barriers such as stigma, lack of education, or inadequate support systems. Understanding how breastfeeding is viewed in various parts of the world provides insight into the diverse challenges and successes in promoting this essential practice.

1. Western Countries: Balancing Modernity and Tradition

In many Western countries, such as the United States, the United Kingdom, and Canada, breastfeeding is recognized as the best option for infant nutrition, yet cultural and practical challenges persist.

a. **United States:** The United States has a mixed approach to breastfeeding. While the American Academy of Pediatrics strongly advocates for exclusive breastfeeding for the first six months, societal attitudes can be ambivalent. Many mothers face pressure to return to work shortly after childbirth, often without paid maternity leave, which can hinder breastfeeding. Public breastfeeding can still attract negative attention, despite legal protections. However, there has been a growing movement to normalize breastfeeding, with public health campaigns and breastfeeding-friendly policies in workplaces and public spaces.

b. **United Kingdom:** The UK has similar challenges, with lower breastfeeding rates compared to other European countries. While breastfeeding is encouraged, especially in public health messaging, many mothers still face societal stigma and lack of support, particularly in lower socio-economic groups. The government has implemented initiatives to promote breastfeeding, but the impact has been uneven across different regions and communities.

c. Canada: Canada has a more supportive environment for breastfeeding, with higher rates of breastfeeding initiation and duration. The country offers paid maternity leave, and public health campaigns actively promote breastfeeding. Public breastfeeding is generally accepted, and there is widespread support from healthcare providers and lactation consultants. However, challenges remain, particularly in remote or indigenous communities where access to support services may be limited.

2. European Countries: Strong Support and High Rates

Many European countries, particularly in Scandinavia, have some of the highest breastfeeding rates in the world, supported by robust public policies and cultural acceptance.

a. Norway and Sweden: Norway and Sweden are often cited as exemplary in their support for breastfeeding. Both countries offer generous parental leave policies, which allow mothers to stay home for extended periods, facilitating exclusive breastfeeding. Public health campaigns are pervasive, and breastfeeding in public is widely accepted and normalized. These factors contribute to very high breastfeeding rates, with most mothers breastfeeding well beyond the first year.

b. France: France presents a contrasting picture. Despite being a developed country, France has relatively low breastfeeding rates. Cultural attitudes in France often favor bottle-feeding, and there is less public and governmental support for breastfeeding compared to other European nations. Many mothers return to work early, and breastfeeding in public is less common and can be viewed as inappropriate. However, recent public health efforts aim to change these perceptions and increase breastfeeding rates.

c. Germany: Germany has moderate breastfeeding rates, with strong initial support but lower long-term breastfeeding. The country provides paid maternity leave and has a growing network of breastfeeding support groups. Public attitudes towards breastfeeding are generally positive, though there is still some discomfort with public breastfeeding.

3. Asian Countries: Tradition Meets Modernity

Breastfeeding practices in Asia vary widely, influenced by traditional beliefs, modernization, and public health policies.

a. Japan: In Japan, breastfeeding is traditionally valued, and most mothers begin breastfeeding immediately after birth. However, Japan's demanding work culture can make it challenging for mothers to continue breastfeeding after returning to work. There is also a strong cultural emphasis on modesty, which can make public breastfeeding less common. The government has implemented policies to support breastfeeding, but social expectations and workplace norms can create barriers.

b. India: In India, breastfeeding is widely practiced and supported by cultural norms. Breastfeeding is often seen as a natural and essential part of motherhood, and extended breastfeeding is common. However, there are significant challenges, particularly in rural areas, where access to healthcare and education about breastfeeding may be limited. Malnutrition and poverty can also impact the ability to breastfeed effectively. The Indian government has launched initiatives to promote breastfeeding, particularly in urban areas where formula feeding is becoming more prevalent.

c. China: China's breastfeeding rates have fluctuated over the years. Traditional Chinese culture strongly supports breastfeeding, but rapid modernization and aggressive marketing of formula have led to a decline in breastfeeding rates, especially in urban areas. The Chinese government has responded with campaigns to promote breastfeeding, and there is a growing awareness of its benefits. However, the pressure of returning to work early and the lack of breastfeeding-friendly workplaces remain significant barriers.

4. African Countries: Cultural Practices and Health Challenges

In many African countries, breastfeeding is the norm, but various challenges, including health crises and socio-economic factors, impact breastfeeding practices.

a. Sub-Saharan Africa: In Sub-Saharan Africa, breastfeeding is almost universal, and cultural norms strongly support it. Extended breastfeeding is common, and breastfeeding in public is generally accepted. However, the region faces significant challenges, including high rates of maternal and infant mortality, malnutrition, and the impact of HIV/AIDS, which can complicate breastfeeding practices. International organizations and governments have worked to promote safe breastfeeding practices, particularly in the context of HIV, where the benefits of breastfeeding must be weighed against the risk of transmission.

b. South Africa: South Africa presents a unique case where breastfeeding rates have been influenced by the HIV epidemic. For years, formula feeding was promoted to prevent mother-to-child transmission of HIV, leading to a decline in breastfeeding. However, with advancements in treatment, there has been a renewed emphasis on breastfeeding as the best option for infant health, and efforts are being made to increase breastfeeding rates through public health campaigns and support services.

5. Latin American Countries: Breastfeeding and Social Support

In Latin America, breastfeeding is generally encouraged, but practices and support levels vary across the region.

a. Brazil: Brazil has made significant strides in promoting breastfeeding through government-led initiatives. The country has implemented the "Baby-Friendly Hospital Initiative," which encourages hospitals to support breastfeeding from birth. Breastfeeding is culturally accepted, and public health campaigns have successfully increased breastfeeding rates. However, socio-economic disparities still affect access to breastfeeding support, particularly in rural and impoverished areas.

b. Mexico: In Mexico, breastfeeding is common, but rates of exclusive breastfeeding are lower than in other Latin American countries. Cultural practices, such as early introduction of solid foods and formula, impact breastfeeding duration. The Mexican government has launched campaigns to promote exclusive breastfeeding, but challenges such as poverty, lack of education, and aggressive marketing of formula persist.

c. Argentina: Argentina has a mixed breastfeeding landscape, with relatively high initiation rates but lower rates of exclusive breastfeeding. Public health initiatives have focused on increasing awareness of the benefits of breastfeeding, but cultural factors, such as the perception of breastfeeding as a private matter, can limit public support.

Conclusion

Breastfeeding practices and attitudes vary widely across the globe, shaped by cultural norms, public policies, socio-economic factors, and health challenges. While some countries have created supportive environments that facilitate breastfeeding, others struggle with barriers that prevent many mothers from breastfeeding successfully. Understanding these global perspectives highlights the importance of culturally sensitive approaches to promoting breastfeeding, recognizing that what works in one country may not be effective in another. To support breastfeeding worldwide, it is essential to address the unique challenges faced by mothers in different cultural and socio-economic contexts, ensuring that all mothers have the resources and support they need to provide the best possible nutrition for their infants.

Section VIII: Considerations for Women When Choosing to Breastfeed

Breastfeeding is a personal decision that every woman must make based on her unique circumstances, values, and preferences. While breastfeeding is widely recognized as the best source of nutrition for infants, it also requires significant commitment and involves various physical, emotional, and practical considerations. When deciding whether to breastfeed, women must weigh several factors, including health benefits, lifestyle, support systems, and personal comfort. Understanding these considerations can help women make informed decisions that are best for both them and their babies.

1. Health Benefits for the Baby

The health benefits of breastfeeding for the baby are among the most compelling reasons for mothers to consider this option. Breast milk is rich in nutrients and antibodies that are crucial for the infant's development and immune system.

a. Nutritional Superiority: Breast milk is perfectly tailored to meet the nutritional needs of the baby, containing the right balance of proteins, fats, vitamins, and minerals. It is easier for the baby to digest compared to formula, reducing the risk of gastrointestinal issues.

b. Immune Support: Breast milk contains antibodies and immune-boosting factors that help protect the baby from infections and illnesses. Studies have shown that breastfed babies have a lower risk of developing respiratory infections, ear infections, and allergies.

c. Long-Term Health Benefits: Breastfeeding has been associated with lower risks of chronic conditions later in life, such as obesity, type 2 diabetes, and certain types of cancer. Additionally, breastfed babies are less likely to develop conditions like asthma and eczema.

2. Health Benefits for the Mother

Breastfeeding also offers significant health benefits for the mother, which should be considered when making the decision.

a. Postpartum Recovery: Breastfeeding helps the uterus contract and return to its pre-pregnancy size more quickly, reducing postpartum bleeding. It also promotes weight loss by burning extra calories.

b. Reduced Risk of Certain Cancers: Women who breastfeed have a lower risk of developing breast and ovarian cancers. The protective effect increases with the duration of breastfeeding.

c. Hormonal and Emotional Benefits: Breastfeeding releases oxytocin, a hormone that promotes bonding between mother and baby and can reduce the risk of postpartum depression. Many women find that breastfeeding fosters a strong emotional connection with their child.

3. Lifestyle and Practical Considerations

The decision to breastfeed also involves practical considerations that can impact a woman's daily life and routines.

a. Time Commitment: Breastfeeding requires a significant time commitment, especially in the early months when feeding is frequent. Mothers need to consider whether they can accommodate the demands of breastfeeding with their other responsibilities, such as work or caring for other children.

b. Flexibility and Mobility: Breastfeeding can limit a mother's flexibility, particularly in the early months when the baby is nursing frequently. Some women may find it challenging to balance breastfeeding with other activities, such as work, travel, or social engagements.

c. Sleep Patterns: Breastfeeding, especially during the night, can affect a mother's sleep patterns. Frequent night feedings can lead to sleep deprivation, which may be a concern for some mothers.

d. Weaning and Transition: Women need to consider their long-term plans for feeding, including how and when they plan to wean the baby from breastfeeding. Some may choose to combine breastfeeding with formula feeding or introduce solids at an earlier stage.

4. Support Systems

The presence of a strong support system can significantly influence a woman's decision to breastfeed.

a. Partner and Family Support: Support from a partner, family members, or close friends can make a significant difference in a woman's breastfeeding experience. Encouragement, assistance with household tasks, and emotional support are crucial during the early stages of breastfeeding.

b. Access to Professional Support: Lactation consultants, healthcare providers, and breastfeeding support groups can provide valuable guidance and assistance. Women should consider whether they have access to these resources, especially if they encounter challenges such as latching difficulties or low milk supply.

c. Workplace Support: For working mothers, the availability of breastfeeding-friendly policies in the workplace is an important consideration. This includes access to private spaces for pumping, flexible work schedules, and supportive employers.

5. Personal Comfort and Preferences

Personal comfort and individual preferences play a critical role in the decision to breastfeed.

a. Physical Comfort: Some women may experience discomfort or pain while breastfeeding, particularly in the early stages. Nipple pain, engorgement, and mastitis are common issues that can affect a mother's comfort and willingness to continue breastfeeding.

b. Body Image and Modesty: Women who are concerned about changes in their body shape or who feel uncomfortable with breastfeeding in public may hesitate to breastfeed. Cultural norms and personal beliefs about modesty can also influence a woman's decision.

c. Emotional Readiness: Breastfeeding is not just a physical activity but also an emotional one. Some women may feel anxious or uncertain about breastfeeding, while others may feel a strong desire to nurture their baby in this way. Emotional readiness and confidence in the ability to breastfeed are important factors to consider.

6. Cultural and Societal Influences

Cultural and societal influences can shape a woman's attitudes towards breastfeeding and impact her decision.

a. Cultural Norms: In some cultures, breastfeeding is the norm and is strongly encouraged, while in others, formula feeding may be more common. Women need to consider how their cultural background and community practices influence their decision.

b. Societal Expectations: Society's attitudes towards breastfeeding, particularly public breastfeeding, can affect a woman's comfort level. In societies where breastfeeding is stigmatized, women may feel pressured to formula feed or to breastfeed only in private.

c. Public Health Campaigns: Public health campaigns and government policies that promote breastfeeding can influence a woman's decision. These campaigns often highlight the benefits of breastfeeding and provide resources to support breastfeeding mothers.

Conclusion

Choosing to breastfeed is a personal decision that involves considering a wide range of factors. Women must weigh the health benefits for themselves and their babies, the practical implications for their lifestyle, the level of support they can expect from family and society, and their own comfort and preferences. By taking the time to reflect on these considerations, women can make informed decisions that align with their values, needs, and circumstances. Ultimately, the choice to breastfeed should be respected and supported, recognizing that every woman's situation is unique.

Section IV: Weaning: How Women Should Transition Their Baby from Breastfeeding

Weaning is a significant milestone in a baby's development and a complex, emotional journey for both mother and child. The process of transitioning a baby from breastfeeding to other forms of nutrition requires careful planning, patience, and sensitivity to the baby's needs. The timing and method of weaning vary widely depending on the mother's and baby's readiness, cultural practices, and individual circumstances. Whether a mother chooses to wean gradually or abruptly, understanding the principles of weaning can help ensure a smooth and positive experience for both.

1. Determining the Right Time to Wean

The decision about when to begin weaning is highly personal and depends on various factors, including the baby's age, developmental readiness, and the mother's needs.

a. Age and Developmental Milestones: The World Health Organization (WHO) recommends exclusive breastfeeding for the first six months of life, followed by continued breastfeeding along with complementary foods up to two years of age or beyond. However, the actual timing of weaning varies. Some babies may show signs of readiness earlier, while others may need more time. Signs of readiness include showing interest in solid foods, being able to sit up and swallow, and losing the tongue-thrust reflex that pushes food out of the mouth.

b. Mother's Readiness: A mother's physical and emotional readiness is also crucial in determining the timing of weaning. Some mothers may need to wean due to medical reasons, returning to work, or simply feeling that it is the right time for both her and her baby. It is important for the mother to feel confident and comfortable with her decision, as weaning can be an emotional process.

c. Baby-Led vs. Mother-Led Weaning: Weaning can be either baby-led, where the baby gradually loses interest in breastfeeding, or mother-led, where the mother initiates the process. Baby-led weaning tends to be more gradual and may be easier for the baby, while mother-led weaning might be necessary when there are external factors like work or health concerns.

2. Gradual Weaning: A Step-by-Step Approach

Gradual weaning is often recommended as it allows both the baby and mother to adjust to the change at their own pace. This approach minimizes stress and helps maintain the emotional bond between mother and child.

a. Start by Dropping One Feeding: The gradual weaning process typically begins by eliminating one breastfeeding session at a time. It is often recommended to start with the feeding that the baby seems least interested in, such as a midday feeding. This allows the baby to adjust to the change without feeling deprived.

b. Replace with a Bottle or Cup: As breastfeeding sessions are reduced, mothers can offer a bottle or cup of expressed breast milk, formula, or whole milk (for babies over one year old) as a substitute. Introducing a cup early can help ease the transition, especially for older babies.

c. Introduce Solid Foods: For babies who are six months or older, solid foods can be introduced as part of the weaning process. Offering a variety of nutritious foods can help meet the baby's nutritional needs as breastfeeding decreases. It's important to introduce new foods gradually and watch for any signs of allergies or digestive issues.

d. Eliminate One Feeding Every Few Days: To avoid engorgement and discomfort, it is advisable to drop one breastfeeding session every few days to a week. This gradual reduction allows the mother's milk supply to adjust naturally and reduces the risk of blocked ducts or mastitis.

e. Night Weaning: Nighttime feedings are often the last to go, as they provide comfort to the baby. When weaning from night feedings, offering a comfort object, like a favorite blanket or stuffed animal, can help soothe the baby. Some mothers find it helpful to have their partner take over nighttime soothing to break the association with breastfeeding.

3. Abrupt Weaning: When Gradual Weaning Isn't Possible

In some cases, gradual weaning may not be an option, and mothers may need to stop breastfeeding more quickly. This could be due to health issues, medication, or other urgent reasons.

a. Managing Discomfort: Abrupt weaning can lead to engorgement, discomfort, and an increased risk of mastitis. To manage this, mothers can express just enough milk to relieve discomfort, use cold compresses, and wear a supportive bra. Over-the-counter pain relievers can also help alleviate discomfort.

b. Emotional Support: Abrupt weaning can be emotionally challenging for both mother and baby. It is important for mothers to seek support from partners, family members, or healthcare providers during this time. Keeping the baby close and offering plenty of cuddles and comfort can help ease the emotional transition.

c. Nutritional Considerations: When abruptly weaning, it is crucial to ensure that the baby receives adequate nutrition from other sources. Consulting a pediatrician to develop a feeding plan that meets the baby's nutritional needs is advisable.

4. Emotional Aspects of Weaning

Weaning is not just a physical transition but also an emotional one. Both mother and baby may experience a range of feelings, from sadness to relief.

a. The Baby's Perspective: Babies often rely on breastfeeding for comfort, security, and bonding. As breastfeeding decreases, babies may seek comfort in other ways, such as through increased cuddling, sucking on a pacifier, or carrying a favorite toy. It's important to be patient and responsive to the baby's emotional needs during this time.

b. The Mother's Perspective: Mothers may experience mixed emotions during weaning. Some may feel a sense of loss or sadness as the breastfeeding relationship ends, while others may feel relief and a sense of freedom. Hormonal changes associated with weaning can also affect a mother's mood, and it's important to be aware of these potential shifts.

c. Maintaining Bonding: Weaning does not mean the end of the bond between mother and child. Continuing to spend quality time together, engaging in skin-to-skin contact, and maintaining routines like bedtime stories can help sustain the emotional connection.

5. Cultural and Social Considerations

Cultural and social factors can influence how and when a mother chooses to wean.

a. Cultural Norms: In some cultures, extended breastfeeding is the norm, and weaning may occur much later, often naturally as the child loses interest. In other cultures, there may be pressure to wean earlier, either due to social expectations or practical considerations.

b. Family and Social Support: The support of family members, particularly partners, can play a crucial role in the weaning process. Involving them in the decision-making and transition process can help ensure a smoother experience.

c. Public Perception: In some communities, breastfeeding beyond a certain age may be viewed negatively, which can influence a mother's decision to wean. Mothers may need to navigate societal pressures and make decisions based on what is best for their child, rather than external opinions.

Conclusion

Weaning is a significant transition that requires thoughtful consideration and planning. Whether gradual or abrupt, the process should be guided by the needs and readiness of both mother and baby. By taking a patient, responsive approach and seeking support when needed, mothers can help ensure that weaning is a positive experience that strengthens the bond with their child. Ultimately, the goal of weaning is to move toward the next stage of development in a way that honors the unique relationship between mother and baby.

Section X: The Dos and Don'ts of Breastfeeding

Breastfeeding is a natural and rewarding experience for both mother and baby, but it can also be challenging, especially for first-time mothers. Knowing the dos and don'ts of breastfeeding can help ensure that both mother and baby benefit from this important practice. This guide provides a comprehensive overview of the key practices to follow and pitfalls to avoid making breastfeeding a successful and enjoyable experience.

The Dos of Breastfeeding

Do Start Breastfeeding Soon After Birth

- **Why It Matters:** Initiating breastfeeding within the first hour after birth is crucial for establishing a successful breastfeeding relationship. This practice, often called the "golden hour," takes advantage of the baby's natural instinct to suckle and helps to stimulate milk production.
- **Tip:** Skin-to-skin contact during this time can also promote bonding and help the baby adjust to life outside the womb.

Do Ensure Proper Latching

- **Why It Matters:** Proper latching is essential for effective breastfeeding. A good latch ensures that the baby can draw enough milk and prevents nipple pain and damage for the mother.
- **Tip:** To achieve a proper latch, make sure the baby's mouth covers most of the areola, not just the nipple. The baby's lips

should be flanged outward, and you should hear a rhythmic sucking and swallowing pattern.

Do Breastfeed on Demand

- **Why It Matters:** Breastfeeding on demand, rather than on a strict schedule, helps to establish and maintain an adequate milk supply. Babies have different feeding needs and allowing them to feed when they are hungry supports their growth and development.
- **Tip:** Look for early hunger cues, such as rooting, sucking on hands, or lip-smacking, rather than waiting for the baby to cry.

Do Stay Hydrated and Eat a Balanced Diet

- **Why It Matters:** Breastfeeding mothers need extra fluids and nutrients to maintain their energy levels and support milk production. Staying hydrated and eating a well-balanced diet rich in fruits, vegetables, whole grains, and lean proteins is essential.
- **Tip:** Keep a water bottle nearby while breastfeeding and try to include nutrient-dense snacks throughout the day.

Do Practice Skin-to-Skin Contact

- **Why It Matters:** Skin-to-skin contact is beneficial for both mother and baby. It helps regulate the baby's body temperature, heart rate, and breathing, and it promotes bonding and milk production.
- **Tip:** Practice skin-to-skin contact not just after birth, but also during feedings and throughout the day, especially in the early weeks.

Do Seek Support and Education

- **Why It Matters:** Breastfeeding can be challenging, and seeking support from lactation consultants, healthcare providers, or breastfeeding support groups can make a significant difference. Education on breastfeeding techniques and what to expect can help mothers overcome common challenges.
- **Tip:** Don't hesitate to reach out for help if you're experiencing difficulties. Early intervention can prevent problems from worsening.

Do Alternate Breasts During Feedings

- **Why It Matters:** Alternating breasts during feedings helps ensure that both breasts are emptied, which supports milk production and prevents engorgement. It also ensures that the baby receives both foremilk (which is lower in fat) and hindmilk (which is richer in fat).
- **Tip:** Start each feeding with the breast that was not used last or use a reminder like a bracelet or hair tie on the wrist of the breast that needs to be used next.

Do Take Care of Your Nipples

- **Why It Matters:** Sore or cracked nipples can make breastfeeding painful and may lead to infection. Proper nipple care is essential for maintaining comfort and continuing breastfeeding.
- **Tip:** Allow your nipples to air dry after feedings and apply lanolin cream or breast milk to soothe and heal the skin. Wear breathable, cotton nursing bras to reduce irritation.

The Don'ts of Breastfeeding

Don't Supplement with Formula Unnecessarily

- **Why It Matters:** Supplementing with formula can interfere with establishing a good milk supply, especially in the early weeks. It can also lead to nipple confusion, where the baby struggles to switch between breast and bottle.
- **Tip:** Unless medically necessary, avoid supplementing with formula in the first few weeks. If you need to supplement, consider using expressed breast milk instead.

Don't Ignore Pain or Discomfort

- **Why It Matters:** Pain during breastfeeding is not normal and can be a sign of an improper latch, infection, or other issues. Ignoring pain can lead to more serious problems, such as mastitis or a decrease in milk supply.
- **Tip:** If you experience persistent pain, seek help from a lactation consultant or healthcare provider to address the underlying issue.

Don't Restrict Feeding Times

- **Why It Matters:** Limiting the time a baby spends at the breast can prevent them from getting the full amount of milk they need, including the fatty hindmilk that comes at the end of a feeding. This can affect their growth and weight gain.
- **Tip:** Allow your baby to nurse for as long as they want on each breast, switching sides when they naturally release the nipple.

Don't Overlook Signs of Hunger or Fullness

- **Why It Matters:** Responding to your baby's hunger cues is essential for their health and well-being. Ignoring these cues can lead to frustration for both mother and baby and can affect milk supply.
- **Tip:** Learn to recognize early hunger cues and signs of fullness. A baby who is full will often release the nipple on their own, appear relaxed, and may fall asleep.

Don't Wean Abruptly Without Planning

- **Why It Matters:** Abrupt weaning can cause physical discomfort, emotional distress, and a risk of mastitis for the mother. For the baby, it can be a difficult adjustment that leads to increased fussiness or difficulty sleeping.
- **Tip:** Plan weaning gradually by slowly dropping one feeding at a time, giving both you and your baby time to adjust.

Don't Rely on Breastfeeding as the Only Form of Birth Control

- **Why It Matters:** While breastfeeding can delay the return of menstruation and reduce fertility, it is not a foolproof method of contraception. Ovulation can occur before the first postpartum period, leading to an unexpected pregnancy.
- **Tip:** If you want to avoid pregnancy, discuss additional contraceptive options with your healthcare provider.

Don't Compare Yourself to Others

- **Why It Matters:** Every mother and baby are different, and what works for one pair may not work for another. Comparing yourself to others can lead to unnecessary stress and feelings of inadequacy.

- **Tip:** Focus on your unique breastfeeding journey and remember that any amount of breastfeeding is beneficial for your baby.

Don't Be Afraid to Breastfeed in Public

- **Why It Matters:** Breastfeeding in public is a normal and natural way to feed your baby. Feeling self-conscious or afraid to nurse in public can limit your ability to go out and enjoy life with your baby.
- **Tip:** Practice nursing in front of a mirror at home to build confidence and use a nursing cover or wear clothes designed for breastfeeding if it helps you feel more comfortable.

Conclusion

Breastfeeding is a journey that requires knowledge, patience, and support. By following these dos and don'ts, mothers can create a positive and successful breastfeeding experience. It is essential to remember that every breastfeeding journey is unique, and what works for one mother and baby may differ for another. The most important thing is to find what works best for you and your baby, ensuring that both of you are healthy, happy, and well-supported throughout the process.

Breastfeeding Resources for Women

Breastfeeding is a rewarding but sometimes challenging journey, and many women benefit from the support and guidance provided by various resources. These resources can help with everything from understanding the basics of breastfeeding to dealing with specific challenges. Here is a summary of the most valuable breastfeeding resources available to women:

1. Lactation Consultants

- **What They Offer:** Lactation consultants are healthcare professionals specializing in breastfeeding. They provide personalized support, helping mothers with latching techniques, managing milk supply, and addressing any breastfeeding challenges.
- **How to Access:** Many hospitals and clinics have lactation consultants on staff. You can also find private lactation consultants through referrals or professional organizations such as the International Lactation Consultant Association (ILCA).

2. Breastfeeding Support Groups

- **What They Offer:** Support groups provide a community for breastfeeding mothers to share experiences, ask questions, and receive encouragement. These groups can be particularly helpful for new mothers looking for peer support.
- **How to Access:** Local hospitals, community centers, and organizations like La Leche League International (LLLI) often host support groups. There are also online support groups and forums where mothers can connect virtually.

3. Healthcare Providers

- **What They Offer:** Obstetricians, pediatricians, and family doctors can provide breastfeeding guidance and support, including addressing medical concerns related to breastfeeding.

- **How to Access:** Regular check-ups and appointments with your healthcare provider are opportunities to discuss breastfeeding and receive advice tailored to your health and your baby's needs.

4. Breastfeeding Hotlines and Helplines

- **What They Offer:** Hotlines and helplines offer immediate assistance for breastfeeding questions or concerns. Trained counselors can provide support on a wide range of issues, from latching difficulties to milk supply concerns.
- **How to Access:** Many organizations, including government health departments and non-profits like the National Breastfeeding Helpline in the U.S., offer these services.

5. Educational Websites and Online Resources

- **What They Offer:** Numerous websites provide educational articles, videos, and resources on breastfeeding. These sites can be a great way to learn more about breastfeeding, find troubleshooting tips, and stay informed about best practices.
- **How to Access:** Reputable sources include the World Health Organization (WHO), the American Academy of Pediatrics (AAP), and La Leche League International (LLLI). Many of these organizations offer comprehensive guides and FAQs on their websites.

6. Breastfeeding Apps

- **What They Offer:** Mobile apps dedicated to breastfeeding offer tools for tracking feedings, managing milk supply, and accessing educational content. Some apps also connect mothers with lactation consultants or support communities.

- **How to Access:** Popular breastfeeding apps include Baby Tracker, Medela Family, and Breastfeeding Central, available on app stores for smartphones and tablets.

7. Books and Literature

- **What They Offer:** There are many books on breastfeeding that provide in-depth information, practical tips, and personal stories. Books can be a valuable resource for mothers looking to deepen their understanding of breastfeeding.
- **How to Access:** Books like "The Womanly Art of Breastfeeding" by La Leche League International and "Breastfeeding Made Simple" by Nancy Mohrbacher are widely available at bookstores, libraries, and online.

8. Breastfeeding-Friendly Workplaces

- **What They Offer:** Employers that support breastfeeding mothers provide accommodations such as private spaces for pumping, flexible work hours, and access to lactation consultants.
- **How to Access:** Discuss your needs with your employer and familiarize yourself with your rights regarding breastfeeding at work. In many countries, there are laws that protect the rights of breastfeeding mothers in the workplace.

9. Government and Non-Profit Programs

- **What They Offer:** Many governments and non-profit organizations offer programs that support breastfeeding, including educational campaigns, financial assistance for breastfeeding supplies, and access to breastfeeding classes.
- **How to Access:** Programs like WIC (Women, Infants, and Children) in the U.S. provide resources and support to low-income mothers. Check with your local health department or community organizations for available services.

Conclusion

Breastfeeding can be a complex journey, but with the right resources, mothers can find the support they need to succeed. Whether through professional lactation consultants, peer support groups, or educational materials, there are numerous ways for women to access help and guidance. Knowing where to find these resources and how to use them can make a significant difference in a mother's breastfeeding experience, ensuring both she and her baby thrive.

Also by LM Glenn

25 Chores for Kids: Teaching Kids Responsibility
After-school Recipes for Kids by Kids
Corny Dad Jokes
Mom to Be: Quick Guide for Breastfeeding
Teaching your Kids Spanish: A Quick How-To Guide

About the Author

LM Glenn is a working mom balancing her faith, career, and family with grace. She deeply values her time with her loved ones, whether at home or cheering together at baseball games, a sport she's passionate about. Her faith guides her daily life, and she finds moments of peace and reflection through prayer and worship. In her downtime, she enjoys reading for pleasure, finding inspiration in both spiritual and fictional works, and unwinding with Netflix binge-watching sessions. Her life is a harmonious blend of faith, family, work, and personal joys, all centered around her love for God and her family.